Burn the Blubber

How to Lose Belly Fat Fast, and For Good!

How To Lose Weight Fast, Keep it Off & Renew the Mind, Body & Spirit Through Fasting, Smart Eating & Practical Spirituality - Volume 4

ROBERT DAVE JOHNSTON

Published by:

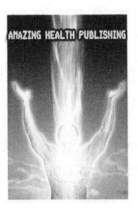

If you are interested in reading new releases, follow Rob on Twitter @FitnessFasting

Copyright

Disclaimer & Legal Notices

The health-related information and suggestions contained in any of the books or written material mentioned above are based on the research, experience and opinions of the Author and other contributors. Nothing herein should be misinterpreted as actual medical advice, such as one would obtain from a Physician, or as advice for self-diagnosis or as any manner of prescription for self-treatment.

Neither is any information herein to be considered a particular or general cure for any ailment, disease or other health issue. The material contained within is offered strictly and solely for the purpose of providing Holistic health education to the general public. Persons with any health condition should consult a medical professional before entering this or any fasting, weight loss, detoxification or health related program. Even if you suffer from no known illness, we recommend that you seek medical advice before starting any fasting, weight loss and/or detoxification program, and before choosing to follow any advice given this book. For any products or services mentioned or suggested in this book, you should read all packaging and instructions, as no substance, natural or drug, can be guaranteed to work in everyone.

Information and statements regarding dietary supplements, products or services mentioned in this book many not have been evaluated by the Food and Drug Administration and are not intended to diagnose, treat, cure, or prevent any disease. Never disregard or delay in seeking professional medical advice because of something you have read in this book.

Nothing that you read in this book should be regarded as medical or health advice. If you do anything recommended in this book, without the supervision of a licensed medical doctor, you do so at your own risk.

Not recommended for persons with any health related condition unless supervised by a qualified health practitioner.

Because there is always some risk involved in any health-related program, the Author, Publisher and contributors assume no responsibility for any adverse effects or consequences resulting from the use of any suggested preparations or procedures described in any of the books or other written materials associated with the website FitnessThroughFasting.com. The author reserves the right to alter and update his opinions based on new conditions at any time.

Dedication

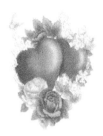

This series of books are dedicated to my mother Sonia Noemi, without whom I would not even be alive today. I love you mom. Thank you for never losing faith in me and supporting me, even when everything seemed hopeless and everyone else had given up on me. I owe you everything. I could collect all of the precious stones on this earth and lay them on your lap, and even still, I would not even come close to giving back to you all that you have given me.

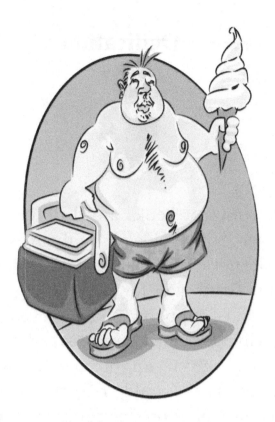

"Yes, I had a very bad case of *'man boobs'* as they call it nowadays. To me, it was disgusting. "

Chapter 1
The Trouble with Flab

Hello and welcome! In this book we are going to talk about something that I get TONS of emails on, and that is losing belly fat. At first I was unsure whether or not to write this as my main expertise is in fasting for weight loss and detoxification. However, since I was overweight for so many years, and since I know how frustrating it can be to lose belly fat, I figured "*what the heck,*" and have written what you are now reading.

Over the years I have gathered a lot of information on the topic, not to mention that I have had to fight <u>my own battle</u> with belly fat. I am certain that, what has worked for me, will also work for you <u>IF</u> you are willing to do what it takes. My goal is to equip you with everything that you need to lose belly fat *'for good.'* Take your time and read this book several times.

It may take you a while to implement all of the suggestions that I give you. If you have been overweight for a long time, or if you have been thin but have had <u>stubborn belly fat</u>, then you will need to be patient and persistent. A lot of people that I work with are educated and of strong will to accomplish anything. However, they are filled with impatience and are **overly-emotional about their weight**. Therefore, they start a weight loss program like gangbusters, but quit a few weeks later because the results they wanted *'did not happen fast enough.'*

Please do not allow this to happen to you. **It will take as long as it will take.** If you can take the *'time'* equation out of your mind and simply take consistent action, you <u>will</u> get there. If, on the other hand, you are constantly weighing yourself and whining about **every little ounce upward or downward on the scale**, then you will struggle.

The 'Screw It' Syndrome

<u>Be as unemotional as possible</u>.

Be methodical and precise. There is no room for emotions in weight loss. They will <u>always</u> suck you dry of motivation and lead you to make foolhardy (*and counterproductive*) decisions. Ever heard of the 'screw *it*' syndrome? Yeah... I sure have. *"Screw it, this is taking too long... screw it, I am tired of waiting,"* and on and on. There are a million ends to that sentence. I'm sure you can come up with a few of your own. Beware of the *"Screw It"* Syndrome. It is <u>always</u> looming and aiming to cut short your weight loss efforts. It is forever seeking for ways to sink you back into poor eating, weight gain and despair.

I tell you all of this because I know very well what it is like to struggle with belly fat (*and flab in general*). I was obese for more than 25 years. Even after I lost the first 110 pounds with different forms of fasting and cleansing diets, it **still took me another 18 months to lose the belly fat**. It is a real pain in the neck, but it <u>**CAN**</u> be vanquished.

I would suggest that, in addition to this book, you also read Volume 1 of the series, **'The Permanent Weight Loss Diet.** That book will support everything that you learn here and provides detailed instructions on a **very effective diet that you can follow**

long-term.

Let's dive right in and take a look at what belly fat is and its effect on health.

Belly Fat Definition

Belly fat sucks. I can't think of another way to put it. If you're reading this book, then you probably agree. It gives us a flabby, wobbly appearance, it is a soft, jelly-like material that accumulates in the abdomen. I don't know about you, but when I had a lot of belly fat, I felt very unattractive.

I would hardly ever take my shirt off because I couldn't stand the way that I looked.

I know that it sounds very superficial, but those were my feelings. I don't think there is anything shallow about wanting to look good. And there is nothing wrong with wanting to get rid of excess belly fat because there is nothing good about it. In my case, the body fat extended to my upper body. Yes, I had a very bad case of *'man boobs'* as they call it nowadays. Oh, it was disgusting.

So, trust me, you are with somebody who has nothing but empathy for your situation.

The best part is that I managed to overcome it and will show you here how I did it. If you are a female, you may also have fat deposits in your thighs, hips and buttocks. All of that can be burned off as well with the information that I will share with you here.

The thing with belly fat is that you don't necessarily have to be fat to have it.

I have many friends who are thin, yet have very large bellies. So, whatever your case may be, I will give you plenty of tips and motivation so that you can solve the belly fat problem <u>once and for all</u>.

It may be hard for you to imagine this right now, but having a flat, sexy belly is <u>very doable</u>. As I said before, all that you need is patience and persistence. If you have that, I am certain that you will achieve tremendous results by putting to practice what I share in this book.

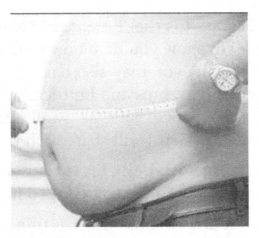

The Omentum

While carrying around a lot of belly fat can make one feel unattractive, what is worse is that it is actually <u>dangerous to your health</u>. Most doctors will tell you that carrying around excess belly fat makes you a candidate for high-blood pressure, diabetes, heart disease and, believe it or not, Alzheimer's.

So even if your motivation now is to look better, I want you to internalize the importance of what you're doing. Losing belly fat, in addition to appearance, has a <u>LOT</u> to do with long-term health. Yes, it is of great importance to take action. Get rid of belly fat <u>NOW</u> so that you don't have to experience health consequences later. You may have heard about the '*omentum*,' the tissue that covers the front of the stomach and down to the liver.

The omentum acts as a '*protective cover*' over the entire abdomen, acting as a '*shield*' or '*bandage*' against inflammation and ruptures as, for example, appendicitis. Having this protective '*canopy*' helps to limit the spread of infection to other parts of the body. The omentum is truly a marvel of the human body. However, people like me who reached levels of morbid obesity, turn the protective omentum into a massive blubber warehouse.

And you don't even have to be obese to have this condition. Excessive fat in the omentum region is what causes the '*pot belly*' or '*beer belly*' look in most men, and in some women - many of which are totally thin elsewhere but have extended bellies that stick outward. Having a large omentum is <u>extremely dangerous</u> because it fosters inflammation that can result in hardening of the arteries, high-blood pressure (*which leads to strokes*) and the dreaded diabetes. I know that I mentioned some of these health hazards before, but I think it is worthwhile to state them again to emphasize the importance (*and urgency*) of what you are doing. I know that you want to look your best. But **belly fat can literally kill**.

If you are already over 45 years of age, the urgency is even greater. Don't listen to those that will tell you how hard it is to lose fat once we get older. I have worked with people in their sixties and even seventies who produced results.

What matters most is your <u>desire</u> and <u>commitment</u> to make the change. It is never easy to change habits and behaviors that have been with us for many years. But it <u>IS</u> possible. Otherwise I would likely be seven-feet under... dead and buried. I am 46 years of age. Yet I continue to work to improve the quality of my health... and I continue to see results. Like I said, commitment and desire are key. If you have that, then half of the battle is already won!

Chapter 2
The Blubber Inside

The first thing I want you to understand is that there are actually different 'types' of fat in the body. I mean, they are all fat. Fat is fat. But fat does accumulate in different places inside the body.

Subcutaneous Fat

This is the flab that is stored <u>directly under the skin</u>. The word 'subcutaneous' literally means 'under the skin.' This is the kind of fat that flops around when you walk or when you run your fingers through your belly. Subcutaneous fat contains <u>blood vessels</u> that feed oxygen into the skin and nerves. Having some fat under the skin is actually good because it acts as 'padding' against trauma. However, excessive amounts cause the skin to tighten and stretch, resulting in stretch marks and cellulite. Fat directly under the skin also acts as a kind of 'energy storage' used when you take part in high-impact/strenuous activities. That is why subcutaneous fat is the first to go whenever you start any kind of weight loss program. Older people sometimes inject fat directly under the skin (*particularly in the face*) to reduce signs of aging and 'fill-in' a gaunt appearance.

Visceral Fat

This is the more dangerous kind of fat because it forms deep inside your body, like packing material in between and around your internal organs. This is also the kind of fat that puts your life at risk of serious disease. If you aren't really overweight but still have a little "*paunch*" around the middle, chances are you probably don't have a large accumulation of visceral fat inside. However, if you are significantly overweight or obese, you likely have large amounts of visceral fat storages, so it is <u>absolutely imperative</u> that you lose it before your health is compromised.

Fat Measuring Devices

If you know that you're fat but have never determined your exact body-fat percentage, then now is the time to do it. There are a number of very easy and low-tech ways to do it as well as super high tech methods. The first (*easiest and fastest*) is to simply go to **This Body Fat Calculator (http://www.bmi-calculator.net/body-fat-calculator)**, input the requested info and then press *'enter.'* I tried that online calculator and it is *'somewhat'* accurate. It will help to give you a general idea of what your body fat percentage is. That's a start. If, on the other hand, you want go get a detailed report, then you will need other instruments like the good ol' hand calipers.

Other fat-measuring methods include X-Ray technology, underwater weighing and what is known as bioelectrical impedance. While simple instruments as calipers can be purchased at most sports stores, higher-tech measuring must be done at a research lab or hospital.

Underwater Weighing

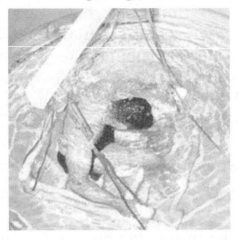

Just like it says, this system works by placing the body fully in water to perform what is known as **hydrostatic weighing**. This is the most precise system that I've even used. I am not too crazy about it because it always tells me that I have more fat than I think. :-(

Seriously, it is a very effective system. If you have the opportunity to get a hydrostatic weighing, go for it. You can call research institutes and hospitals in your area and ask if they do it or know where it is done. The premise of hydrostatic weighing is that muscle is denser than fat, and that fat always pushes to the surface. In other words, fat floats. Therefore, if you have more fat than muscle, then your body will be lighter when immersed in water. It's really awesome. You should look into it and try to find a hydrostatic weighing facility in your area.

Bioelectrical Impedance Analysis

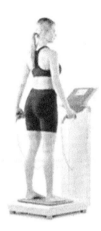

Bioelectrical impedance analysis measures body fat using <u>electric currents</u>. BIA scales run a current through the body. Since muscle has more water than fat, the electric current hits greater resistance when it encounters fat tissue.

The fat percentages are determined based on how the current travels through the body. A BIA scale is also able to measure the percentage of water that you have in your body at any given time. I really can't say much more about BIA because I've never used it. But I have heard that it is indeed quite accurate. Most sports medicine clinics today have one of these devices.

Skinfold Calipers

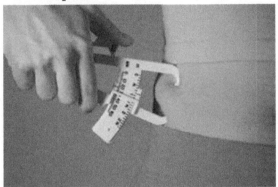

The Skinfold caliper is a scissor-like instrument used to measure the thickness of a layer of skin and fat. In short, it is used to measure how much blubber there is under the skin.

Calipers, in essence, will help you to calculate how much subcutaneous fat (*fat under the skin*) you have. The measurements are added into an equation that then predicts your body density and percentage of body fat. Calipers are the most common way to measure body fat. Even though many people do it by themselves, I recommend that you have a friend do it for you so that you can get the most precise measurements. You'll need to measure fat in <u>three</u> areas of the body.

For men, the measurements should include the thigh, chest and abdomen. For women, test the **waist, triceps and thighs**. The measurements are then added into a special formula to determine the body fat figures.

The most common formula is the **Jackson Pollock 7 Caliper Method.** A quick web search will take you to tons of sites where you can input the information from your measurements into the equation and receive your body fat numbers. If you find yourself struggling with the calipers (*I know that I did at first*) do a YouTube search for *'How to Use Skinfold Calipers.'* You'll get tons of good demonstrations.

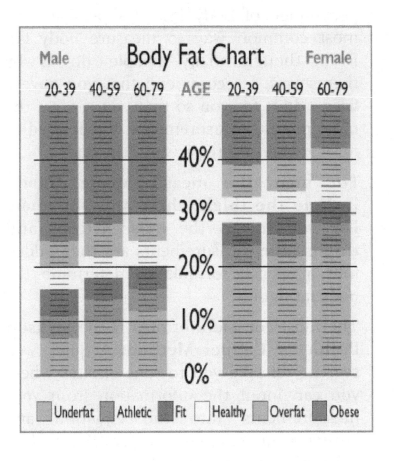

What the Numbers Mean

Determining what your body fat percentage is will give you a solid number that you can work with. Every two weeks, as you continue to work to lose belly fat, you can do another caliper measure and compare. It is amazing when we see fat percentages start to drop. Do you know what your number means?

Your body fat percentage is simply the percentage of fat that your body has at a given time.

If, for example, you are a 46 year-old female who weighs 180 pounds and has 33% body fat, it means that your body has 59.4 pounds of fat (*this is where the belly fat is*) and 120.6 pounds of what is known as lean body mass (*blood, muscle, bones, skin, tissues etc...*)

You would barely fall under the *'healthy range,'* but would probably look and feel better if you reduced body-fat levels to the low 20's.

You still would have plenty of fat to help the body regulate a variety of functions. However, excess fat (*particularly belly fat*) would be little to nonexistent. If you fell under the '*obese*' category, please don't feel bad. You are here taking steps to resolve the problem. Rome was not built in a day, but it **<u>WAS BUILT!</u>**

Continue to move forward with me and give yourself a pat on the back for having the **courage and willingness to confront fat once and for all.**

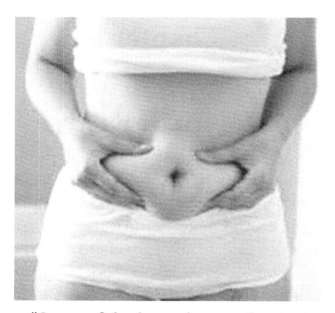

"Some of the latest *'spot reduction'* machines are supposed to be scientifically proven to work. You can sit in the couch watching TV all day with the gadget humming around your belly, burning the fat and making you thin. But what about the person's bad eating habits? The person is left with <u>ZERO</u> tools to stay healthy and lean."

Chapter 3
Spot Reduction:
Myth or Fact?

There are many *'weight loss'* methods out there that talk about losing *'belly fat'* specifically. In other words, targeting the fat stored in the belly exclusively with specific exercises and other gadgets. To be honest with you, I think it's a <u>bunch of baloney</u> designed to take people's money and not much more.

Some of the latest *'spot reduction'* machines are supposed to be <u>scientifically proven</u> to work. You can sit in the couch watching TV all day with the gadget humming around your belly, burning the fat and making you thin. What about the person's bad eating habits? Lazy, inactive lifestyle? What will happen if the gadget breaks, is stolen or lost? The person is left with **<u>ZERO</u>** tools to stay healthy and lean.

This fat loss business is something that we need to do *'the old fashioned way.'* That is the **<u>ONLY</u>** way that you are guaranteed lasting results, as well as the ability to overcome unhealthy lifestyle and eating habits. **If nothing changes, nothing changes**. Strapping a machine to the belly may be alright as a supplement, but the claims that *'this is all you need'* (in my opinion) are misleading.

Here's the truth that I have found in the past 12 years:

There is no such thing as spot reduction.

I believe in **<u>FAT LOSS</u>**. Following a program that reduces my overall levels of body fat... period. I want you to look at this fat loss process as one of <u>reshaping your entire body</u>.

Losing fat **THROUGHOUT** the body, <u>including the belly</u>. That is the best and most effective way to lose fat. I have seen it in myself countless times. And I've seen it in others that I have coached over the years.

Doing 1.000 sit-ups a day to *'burn the belly fat'* doesn't work. I did it. I did it for a **LONG** time. My stomach got hard. Really hard. But the belly fat and *'man boobs'* remained. I needed to cut calories and increase activity so that **MY ENTIRE BODY** would start to shed fat. I clarify this now because I am not here to give you *'miracle cures'* or unrealistic expectations. The tips and suggestions that I am going to give you work **IF** you are willing to roll up your sleeves and do some work. If, on the other hand, you are looking for some *'instant fat loss'* system, then throw away this book or give it to somebody else.

What About Fat Loss Pills?

The issue of whether or not to take some kind of *'fat loss'* pill is something else that I am often asked. There is so much garbage out there; thousands upon thousands of products claiming to help you burn fat and give energy.

Sadly, the majority of these products (*none of which are approved by the Food and Drug Administration*) are packed with stimulants like caffeine, ephedrine and other trash. I saw a documentary some time ago that showed a group of *'business men'* creating a weight loss pill with caffeine, ephedrine and flour. Yes... flour as in flour to bake bread. The stimulants are mixed with the powder, stuck inside colorful tablets and voila! Ready for the sales floor, right? I have tried dozens of weight loss/fat burner pills. None of them helped to curb my appetite. Most did give me energy of course because of the caffeine and ephedrine. Fat loss? Zero... nada. After one month of consistent use, there was **NO** difference in my body fat levels. The <u>ONLY</u> supplement that **HAS** shown me fat loss results is called *Chromium Picolinate.*

Chromium Picolinate is a nutritional mineral that helps the body utilize insulin more effectively. It has gained popularity in recent years because of its manifold benefits, including mood stabilization, energy enhancement, acne prevention and.... you guessed it, fat burning and weight loss. I am **SUPER** skeptical about all products that are said to help *'burn fat and reduce appetite.'*

But I must say that, after taking 200 mcg daily of chromium picolinate for two weeks, I noticed that I was eating less and - consequently - getting thinner. The nighttime blinding cravings were notably reduced, and I stopped waking up at 3AM ready to raid the refrigerator.

I work out regularly and follow a very strict diet, so I can't say that this happened by '*magic*.' But, of all of the weight loss/fat burning products out there, chromium picolinate is the only one that ever benefited me.

Recently, the supplement has been marketed as a safe option to steroids because, it is claimed, it can increase strength and lean muscle mass. From my personal experience I would say that this is not so.

While chromium picolinate did help me to eat less and lose some weight, I did not notice any strength-increase benefits. Since chromium picolinate is a nutritional supplement and not a prescription drug, the Food & Drug Administration doesn't investigate the veracity or falsehood of advertisers' claims. In addition, there is no concrete scientific research supporting that chromium picolinate fosters weight loss. My remarks and experiences with this supplement are therefore arbitrary.

Chapter 4
Belly Fat Causes & Solutions

Now I want to start naming the various causes of belly fat and offering you direct tips, strategies and solutions. From now on, each new chapter will present one specific cause for belly fat.

I will explain the cause, give some examples and then give you ways to overcome it. But you have to be good and patient with yourself. This task **CAN** be done and you **WILL** do it. You will need to treat yourself as you would a dear friend that is going through a challenging transition in his or her life. Treat yourself as you would treat that person.

Maybe you have been overweight for many years... maybe you gained a lot of weight recently due to a stressful situation, pregnancy or just a relapse into poor eating habits.

Whatever the case may be, **put away the hammer and stop bashing yourself over**

the head. Putting yourself down for gaining weight (*or being overweight*) will do <u>NOTHING</u> to help you get rid of belly fat. I think that the fact that you are reading this book shows that you realize that you need to make changes, particularly in the way that you eat. But there are many other reasons apart from eating which contribute to increases in belly fat.

I can write hundreds of pages about **Body Mass Index** and calories eaten versus your height and health. You'd probably be snoring in five minutes and never read this book again.

So I want to be practical and to-the-point without getting into a lot of scientific data that I'm sure you already know. I want to give you steps and solutions to the belly fat problem.

We're going to talk about habits and lifestyle. We're going to talk about our bodies as well as the way we eat, think and behave. We have to look at every area that is touched by belly fat. More than anything, what I want is for you to start to lose inches of fat as quickly as possible.

Chapter 5
The Stressful Life

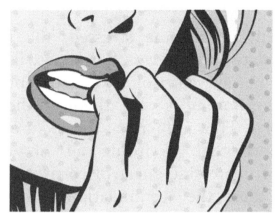

This is another topic that we could write volumes about. You know what stress is: There are only 24 hours in one day and often it feels like it simply isn't enough time to get everything done.

Pressures at home, finances, work... life in general is stressful. With the advent of technology, the Internet and *'instant'* everything, it seems that we are under pressure to do more, and do it faster. But the truth is that, while technology has evolved very rapidly in the past decade, human beings have remained pretty much the same for centuries. Wanting to stay on top of this incessant <u>rat race</u> can cause anyone to get stressed. And, when stressed, most of us tend to eat more (*graze*). Excess body fat is the result.

When we become stressed, the body is inundated with stress hormones, including one named cortisol. Cortisol and other *'stress hormones'* are there to help you survive. They are part of the *"fight or flight"* instinct that is inside all of us. The unfortunate side-effect of cortisol is that it can cause the accumulation of fat in the midsection.

This wouldn't be such a big deal if you only got stressed occasionally, but like many people today, you may experience frequent, prolonged periods of chronic stress, and that can do a number on your body over time. Do you bite your nails? Do you go through periods of intense fear and anxiety about your life and future? Do you have trouble sleeping through the night?

How many times nightly do you get up to use the bathroom, eat, smoke or just stare at the roof and count sheep? If any of these pertain to you, then you are definitely stressed. I myself was a stress monster. I bit my nails to the bare skin, would frequently binge to '*medicate*' my feelings, woke up every two hours at night to urinate, smoke and eat, was plagued with fear, depression, anxiety, negativity ... I was a total catastrophe.

So I understand that stress is very real and that it <u>DOES</u> have a direct impact on body fat. Not only because of the cortisol levels, but because by instinct we tend to eat and drink more when we are stressed. It is a survival mechanism that exceeds its function and can easily become a highly-destructive force in our lives. We need to address this, and we need to make changes in lifestyle right away to counteract it.

Learning to Take it Easy

It may sound a bit farfetched, but if you can learn to relax and not take life so seriously, that in itself will help to start reducing the belly fat. Amazing, huh? No matter what you may be going through, it will pass and come to a resolution regardless of how much you worry and obsess over it. As I was telling you, I was a very high-strung person in my past life. When I say *'past life,'* I mean when I was obese, not some other reincarnation. Everything was a drama to me. Life was a never ending soap opera. I took everything seriously and as a personal affront to **ME**. Fear, anxiety, anger and sadness were my constant companions. I was an emotional basket case.

Since losing 110 pounds and learning to overcome binge eating disorder, I have come to realize that life is simply too short to be a daytime drama. It is what it is. I do the best that I can each moment of every day, and the rest is not in my control. People, places and things have a *'mind'* of their own.

Control Freak

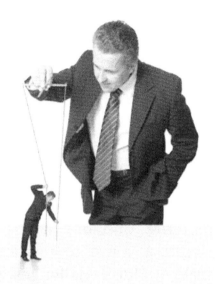

Me trying to control, no matter how hard, <u>always</u> ends up in disaster. So I surrender. I refuse to carry the weight of the world on my shoulders. I have learned to relax and take it easy. That doesn't mean that I neglect my responsibilities. It simply means what I said before:

'I do the best that I can, and surrender the results and timing to God and the universe.'

When I start to feel overwhelmed, I stop

and look at my feet. *"Robert, here are your feet. <u>This</u> is where you are and you cannot be or do <u>anything</u> else <u>except</u> what you are doing <u>right now</u>."* I breathe deep several times and visualize all of the stress and negativity being released with each exhalation. And it works. My initial instinct is to EAT, but I have trained myself to delay the gratification and walk through the feeling instead. Life has become much simpler for me since then.

Stress levels have gone way down and so has my spare tire. I no longer nibble incessantly as I used to as a way to 'medicate' the stress and deal with life's challenges. Bottom line:

I don't medicate my emotions with food anymore.

I walk through my feelings without having to '*fix*' them with food. I am on the road to maturing emotionally which, in turn, has helped me to develop much-needed discipline to simply say **<u>NO</u>**. I don't care how much my body screams and yells and kicks and screams for food.

NO is always the answer. I take action to

resolve the issues in my life WITHOUT using food as a crutch. That alone has been HUGE to help me to get rid of the belly fat. And it will do the same for you.

Acceptance is The Answer

At this point many people ask me: "*Yes, but how can you minimize stress when you can't eliminate the <u>causes</u> of stress?*" Perhaps you have a high-pressure job, or your children are demanding and leave you dragging your elbows on the ground at the end of each day.

Or maybe you are being hit by a number of other stressors in your life. And they all need to be addressed quickly right? You certainly can't leave everything and go to a mountain to chant and meditate. So how can anyone overcome stress under these circumstances?

The answer is simple -. **<u>ACCEPTANCE</u>**. A passage from the book **Alcoholics Anonymous** puts it this way:

"*And acceptance is the answer to all my problems today. When I am disturbed, it is because I find some person, place, thing, or situation - some fact of my life - unacceptable to me, and I can find no serenity until I accept that person, place, thing, or situation as being exactly the way it is supposed to be at this moment. Nothing, absolutely nothing happens in God's world by mistake. Until I could accept my alcoholism, I could not stay sober; unless I accept life completely on life's terms, I cannot be happy. I need to concentrate not so much on what needs to be changed in the world as on what needs to be changed in me and in my attitudes."*

Simple but very powerful truth.

If we live our lives '*waiting*' until everything is *fine and dandy* before we start to let go of stress, it will <u>never</u> happen. There is always some '*new*' situation challenging our emotions. *Life is always full of challenges.* We can't '*wait*' for everything to be alright. No.

We have to come to the point where we <u>accept things exactly as they are</u> <u>at this time and place</u>, <u>AND</u> (*more importantly*) learn to be at ease <u>REGARDLESS</u> of them. This is a mental muscle that takes some time to develop.

But it IS possible to develop it and very necessary. Seriously, managing stress is not about radically changing your life circumstances so you can feel calm. Rather, it is about **learning how to handle stress in healthier ways**.

Certainly, if there are situations that are making you feel pressured and unhappy and you are able to release them, go for it. Unhealthy or dysfunctional relationships, jobs that drain the life out of you, and excessive obligations that can be rescheduled or let go completely are stress factors that you CAN control. Do what is within your grasp to do, and let go of the rest.

Practice constant acceptance and learn NOT to react to everything that you feel. Learn to let crap slide off your back like oil! When I started to do this, the results were drastic and almost instantaneous. I ditched my daily donut trip, which I normally did in the afternoons when I would have the accustomed *'sinking spell.'* Instead of eating five donuts, I went for a 15-minute walk and drank water. And so the miracle began to happen and the belly fat started to diminish.

The bottom line is this: You aren't a <u>VICTIM</u> of circumstances. You are a <u>VICTOR</u> who walks tall <u>IN SPITE</u> of them! I don't say this lightly just to fill space. I mean it. You <u>CAN</u> overcome stress. You <u>CAN</u> learn to walk through each moment of your life with relative peace. Notice that I said *'relative'* peace. That is because there are always ups and downs. We aren't robots. We feel. We feel strongly. And that is a good thing. But let's not allow our *'feelings'* to control us and lead us to become emotionally ill. Let's not allow emotions, circumstances, people, places and things to lead us to *'eat our way'* through life. If you can internalize any truth that I give you, this is one of the most important ones.

Reduce stress, improve the way you manage your thoughts and emotions, and (I guarantee you), the belly fat will start to vanish - very quickly! Why? Because you will find yourself eating less and saying **<u>NO</u>** to the trash foods that beckon you during the day.

You will become a person who takes action to address the daily situations that life offers you, but you will stop reaching for food as the solution to your problems. You will no longer be a puppet, reacting to everything that happens outside of you (*and that you can't control anyway*). *You will start to master your emotions and behaviors.* We never 'graduate,' by the way. We will be learning for as long as we live. But at least we will be making '*new*' mistakes in our lives and moving on to other challenges. We won't get stuck in the same rut over and over. That's the key dear friend.

Annoyance

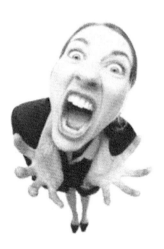

Before I move on to another cause of belly fat and the solution, I want to talk about something that can easily become a plague in our lives ... and that is petty annoyances.

A lot of times, in the past, I didn't necessarily eat because of catastrophic or monumental stress, but because I was annoyed at the reality of life and the inconveniences that I had to face from day to day. The slightest surge in traffic would send me a rage. Line at the bank? I was enraged and full of resentment at the other folks who got there before me. If I was watching TV and commercials interrupted, I would react with anger at *"those scumbag and greedy network executives."* I was always annoyed. Life annoyed me. I annoyed myself. So I ate some more 'to feel better.' Everything that I did was criticized sharply by an internal voice of condemnation. Forgot your keys? *"You're a useless idiot!"*

Somebody was delayed for a few minutes to a meeting? I hated them! And on and on and on I went. Always annoyed by everything; <u>like a little child demanding that the world and everything in it function</u>

the way I wanted it to function **OR ELSE** it was all a conspiracy to inconvenience and upset me. How the heck did I ever live this way? I don't know. No wonder I was stressed and full of anxiety! No wonder I was always eating and had **HUGE** amounts of belly fat!

If you look at all of the things I have mentioned here, <u>NONE</u> of them have to do with adversity. They all have to do with daily life and the things we all deal with. But I didn't accept anything. I was annoyed at all times. Overcoming this monster was tricky but immensely helpful. Today I take a deep breath and smile when I feel annoyance creeping up.

I had to stop being so darn self-centered.

We're all in the same boat. We are all doing the best what we can in life. When I realized that, I started to reach out to others through the day. With a kind word, a smile, letting them go ahead of me in line... *'blessing'* the person that cut me off in traffic instead of spouting obscenities that nobody hears but me. I was always eating because I was always annoyed. I was **'eating <u>AT</u> the world**.' Today I have a lot more friends and I choose to spend more of my day laughing. I laugh at myself, my mistakes and I smile at others and show them kindness.

When I get home at night, <u>rarely</u> do I enter wanting to raid the fridge. It is a much better and decent way to live. Not just because I treat others better, but because I treat MYSELF better. It all starts with the relationship that I have with myself. If my relationship with me sucks, then so will every other relationship that I have. But when I stop bashing myself over the head for the slightest infraction and am kind and patient with ME, then that inevitably spills out in the way that I act with others. And ALL of this affects our eating habits because;

HOSTILE EMOTIONS NEARLY-ALWAYS LED ME TO OVEREAT OR EAT POORLY.

I ate impulsively to soothe the emotional whirlwind in which I was caught.

Let me ask you: Are you angry a lot? Do you find that almost everything upsets you?

Let's be honest: Daily life is full of annoyances. Loud noises, traffic, lines, in-laws... rude and obnoxious clerks, red tape, politicians, the power bill, lousy cable service, slow Internet speed and computers, the government, war, rumors of war, inflation, gas prices, pollution, global warming... you name it. It can all get under our skin **IF** we let it. Starting today, I want you to learn how to <u>let it slide</u>. Imagine that you're covered in oil and that all of that stuff just glides right off of you. I mean, how important is it to react? I am of the belief that things happen for a reason. If I am in a hurry and get stuck behind *'the coupon lady'* at the grocery store, I no longer shoot blood out of my eyes. Instead I ask: "*What is there for me here?*" How do I know that God or *'the universal mind'* isn't leading me to something better, or protecting me from something bad? I really don't know. But when I let go of my anger and focus on <u>living that moment exactly the way that it is</u>, everything begins to flow like magic and all anger evaporates. Give it a shot. You'll be amazed.

Most chronic stress begins as an

underlying feeling of aggravation, frustration, or annoyance.

It's subtle at first, but if you don't diffuse it early on, it will keep snowballing until your heart is racing, your hands are clammy, and your shoulders feel like the Great Wall of China. <u>Pay attention to how you feel throughout the day</u>. This type of self-monitoring is not easy at first, especially if you've never done it before. But it will make your days much less stressful.

My Annoyance Test

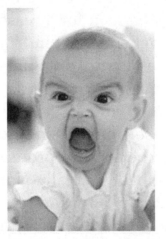

Let me end with something that happened to me last week. A friend and I made a hotel reservation so we could attend a martial arts exhibition up north. We left late and ended up driving at night. I was tired and cranky because I hadn't gotten much sleep the night before. I struggled to drive. I had to stop and drink some coffee, which made me jittery.

The trip was starting to brew into a major annoyance. I was looking forward to getting to the hotel and going to bed. After getting slightly lost, we finally pulled into the hotel entrance. There was a trash can directly in front overflowing with smelly garbage. That really annoyed me because I was told that the hotel *'was new and clean.'*

Rather than make a fuss, I chose to disregard it and go to the front desk to get my key and pass out. The clerks' attire was wrinkled and disheveled and they just stared at me with blank faces. That annoyed me as well because I felt I deserved a smile after that long drive.

I caught my urge to lash out and ignored it.

I smiled and showed them kindness even though I wanted to unload my frustration, tell them about the trash in the front and of their bad manners for not smiling at me and welcoming me.

Turns out, the room they gave me was '*used*.' When I opened the door, the bed was unmade and towels were scattered everywhere. I felt trickles of steam starting to come out of my ears. Let me be blunt: **I was pissed off!** I wanted <u>DESPERATELY</u> to lash out. But, <u>AGAIN</u>, I chose not to. I chose to believe that there was a '*good*' behind all of this. I went back to the same clerks and told them that the room was not clean. They apologized and gave me the key to another room. When I opened the door to the second room, my face was smacked with hot, steamy air. <u>The A/C was broken</u>.

So, once more, I wheeled all of my stuff down the hall to the front lobby. On my way there, **I realized that I had two choices**. I could make a scene and feel justified, or try to get what I wanted: the suite I paid for with a clean bed and a nice air conditioner.

When I went back to the desk, before saying anything about the room, I asked the clerk about her day, commenting that it looked like they all had had a long day. She said that, yes, a convention had come through and that they had been swamped and understaffed. I told her that the day was almost over, that I appreciated she was still there, and that she was doing a good job. Her eyes opened real wide as if she had never heard those words before.

I repeated the same to the other clerks, and then explained that the A/C was broken in the room they gave me. Not only did they give me another room, but it was bigger, nicer and even had a lake view! They carried my luggage upstairs and, from then on, were my best friends and gave me amazing service. Before, I would have become their enemies and felt totally justified. And, given, perhaps the service was not initially what it '*should*' have been.

Is life 'ever' what it 'should' be?

But I didn't want to be '*right*' as much as I wanted a nice room to rest. I looked at them as human beings, not as objects to give me what I needed... and I ended up having a great weekend, not overeating and feeling great. I would have <u>NEVER</u> done that before. I would have spent the weekend thinking about those *"lousy, inefficient clerks and crappy hotel,"* and quite likely eating all types of trash to calm my anger. I would have been stressed out to the max.

It's not about what happens, it's about how we choose to see and respond to the daily situations in our lives.

Chapter 6
Getting Active

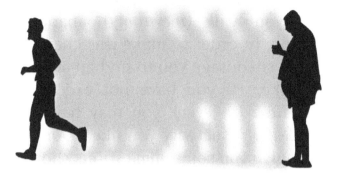

I know that you knew I was going to talk about the often dreaded 'e' word - exercise. I wish I could tell you that you can sit on the couch with the remote control and lose weight by magic. Well, I guess if you eat very little that could possibly happen.

But the fastest way to get rid of belly fat for good is to <u>adopt an active lifestyle</u>. The problem with exercise is that it is typically equated with pain, discomfort, bad times, suffering etc.

What mental association do you have with exercise? The good news is that, it isn't about working out - per se. It's about **finding an activity that you enjoy and**

that brings you pleasure and you can do frequently. If exercising is something that you dislike and do by sheer force of will, the time will come when the willpower will fade and you will (*inevitably*) abandon the routine. In order to make this change last, I highly encourage you to find <u>an activity that you like</u>. If you have not exercised in a long-time (*or ever*), you may have no clue what (*if any*) activity you like. Don't worry. I will give you some suggestions shortly.

There are some very powerful reasons why becoming more active is in your best interest. Number one, of course, you will burn more calories and start to shed belly fat. Secondly, you will find yourself feeling much calmer all around. That, in turn, will help you to say <u>NO</u> to junk food (**or any other food temptation**) when the urge hits.

As we've already seen, the tendency is always to eat poorly (*make bad food choices*) when we are stressed or otherwise emotionally strung out. Exercise, in truth, is the natural drug that brings it all into focus. I'm sure you've heard of the **endorphins**;

the body's <u>natural</u> relievers of pain. Endorphins have an opiate-like effect which fosters a sense of tranquility and wellbeing. Whatever trial or challenging situation you may be going through, you will be able to confront and solve it much faster (and better) if you exercise and give the endorphins a chance to do their job. Before making any important decision, I always like to exercise and give myself time to focus.

The endorphins are amazing. I can be stressed one moment, angry, wanting to eat a dozen cheeseburgers. If I stop, go exercise for 15-30 minutes, 99.9% of the times the negative emotions and urges have disappeared. In 100% of the cases I feel better, clearer and able to make the best possible decisions for myself.

And, honestly, what I put and not put in my mouth is one of the most consequential decisions I can learn to make, don't you think?

I am sure that you understand what I'm talking about and have probably heard it all before. What we need to do now is move you from knowing to doing.

Start at The Beginning

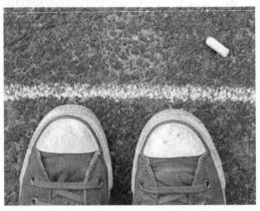

I know that the above subtitle sounds like an oxymoron, but it clearly expresses the point I want to make here. What can you do if you are out of shape, overweight and have never been active? I know what it's like to be in this position.

Staring at the mirror and seeing rolls and rolls of belly fat. Feeling like weight loss is an impossible and insurmountable task. Many people get stuck in this state of overwhelm and never take action.

But you're not going to let that happen, right? Right! Here's what I want you to do:

Start from the beginning... begin from where you are. Huh? I know that sounds silly. But it's true. I have spoken to scores of individuals about exercise and always ask them <u>what keeps them from doing it</u>. The answer is nearly always:

> *"Well, I'm in very bad shape. I'm fat. I wouldn't be able to lift or do much."*

My answer is always: "*Yes, that's true and that's great.*" Great? How on earth is it '*great*' to be weak and out-of-shape? Well, you may not be able to do '*much,*' but you still can do '*something.*' It's amazing how the mind can trick us.

How can anyone who has not been active or exercised expect to be able to do a full triathlon? It simply isn't possible, right? Well, many people who want to lose belly fat don't take action because they feel that unless they can sprint a mile, lift 200 pounds and look thin and sleek overnight, then they might as well not do it at all. Have you ever found yourself thinking that? If not, then you're lucky.

I know good people who have every reason

in the world to lose the belly fat. But they still do nothing because they're *"ashamed that they're so fat and in such bad shape."* **Here's another oxymoron**: The only way to climb a mountain is to start at the bottom (*unless you parachute from a plane*). It doesn't matter how heavy you are, how many times you have tried to lose belly fat before and failed, or whether you have never worked out or been active.

You STILL can make it. Start exactly where you are. You don't need to do a triathlon or be a super athlete to receive the benefits. I remember a man that was 350 pounds overweight. At first all he could do was stand up from the couch and sit down again. He would do ten of those... rest, and then do ten more. That went on for three weeks before he was able to start to actually walk.

HE STARTED FROM WHERE HE WAS AND BUILT FROM THERE.

And, as of today, he has lost the weight and kept it off. He actually is practicing to become a professional cyclist. What would have happened if he had stayed in the couch because he wanted to go straight to cycling? Probably, he'd still be in the couch... or maybe he'd be dead.

<u>Here's the bottom line:</u>

It is <u>urgent</u> for you to find an activity that you enjoy and start to take action, even if at first it is only for five minutes. We don't have time to waste. To lose the belly fat, you **MUST** start to develop a lifestyle that is conducive to the long-term weight loss you desire.

That **IS** what you want, right? You may cringe now – especially if you have never been active. But, I guarantee you, a few months after you get started, you will wonder why you didn't do it before.

Let's be honest here: The only people that don't take part in any activity are those who are dead. If you're still breathing – check your pulse – then you **ARE** alive! You're life is **NOT** meant so that you could grow cobwebs in your arms and legs or get *"thumb strain"* from the remote control or *"couch sores"* on your backside! You're here to live, explore, run, walk, laugh, enjoy... experience **<u>EVERYTHING</u>** that life has to offer! Are you ready? This is <u>YOUR</u> time! Your hour of breakthrough and transcendence!

Choosing Your Activity

So where to start? The sky is the limit. Your choice of activities can be anything from archery to square dancing. What about keeping it very simple ... start walking! All that matters is that you find something that you enjoy. That way you are more likely to keep doing it. **Here's a list of hobbies you may wish to consider:**

Exercise Photography - Taking photos of things you like to look at. If you're reading this page then chances are you have a computer, so digital photography can be a great and rewarding hobby. The best part is that you get to walk around taking photos, and walking is called exercise.

Bird Watching for Weight Loss - Go to your local park and count the birds. Take some of that white bread you're not allowed to eat and feed the birds with it! Looking up into the trees or onto the neighborhood roof tops will stretch those neck muscles, and walking is the best form of exercise yet.

Window Shopping - What could be better than walking around town for an hour or so, looking into the windows of your favorite stores? Everybody likes to shop and everyone likes to dream of what they could buy if money was no object. How about window shopping for the new clothes you will buy when you are thinner?

Flying a Kite – Most of us loved flying kites as kids, why not as we get older?

Sightseeing - You don't have to travel across state or out of the country to go sightseeing. Chances are there are plenty of things going on in your area.

With a little research, you will find events and places to go to that will cost little or no money. Better yet, take a stroll around your neighborhood and look at it from the eyes of a tourist. You'll burn calories and notice a few interesting things at the same time.

Gardening – If you have been out of shape for a long time, then one activity that can help get you going is what is known as gardening for fitness. Stretching down, pulling a few weeds, digging, carting dirt are excellent and help keep the joints working. If you don't have a garden yourself, your local city council probably has a parks and/or gardens program that could use a few volunteers.

Don't Like any of these? Ok, how about:

Badminton - Boxing - Body Building - Camping - Cardio-Workout - Croquet - Fencing - Fishing - Golf - Hiking - Horseback Riding - Hunting - Ice Skating - Inline Skating - Kayak-and-Canoeing - Martial Arts - Pilates - Running - Sailing - Skiing - Snowboarding - Swimming - Tennis - Wakeboarding - Waterskiing - Weight Training - Yoga

One that I found interesting is called **aerobic housecleaning**. No, I'm not kidding. Housework at a moderate level of exertion can burn up as many as 300 calories per hour. So, I ask you: Who needs a gym or expensive equipment when our vacuums, mops, and dust cloths can do the job? Add your favorite music and dance while you clean, and it's not so bad.

Even small activity-increases, over time, will add up!

Take the stairs instead of the elevator. Get off the bus early and walk that last block. Park further away from the store and walk in. Wash your own vehicle instead of taking it to the car wash. A lot of little things can make a **HUGE** difference.

You need to get off the couch my friend.

And, even if you are already active, **we have to increase activity levels even more to get the belly-fat furnace burning**.

Like I said, you don't have to become a super athlete or do **HUGE** amounts of exercise. Just a small increase in your daily activity level will do wonders to help you lose belly fat.

Most people struggle with their weight and health for years for two primary reasons: **lack of discipline and procrastination**.

"Oh yeah, I want to do this or that". But they never get around to it. They start walking each morning but then it rains, so they

don't go that day or the next, or the next, or the next. They start a diet and vow to stick to it. **BUT**, they find that piece of cake, pizza, cheeseburger... whatever *"too tempting"* and fall back into old habits.

They are always starting but never finishing. They are always wishing but never achieving. They are always longing for something but never rouse the courage to do it.

The good news is you can still do it. No matter how many times you have tried and failed before, you <u>CAN</u> lose the belly fat and feel better in the process.

Chapter 7
Silence is Golden

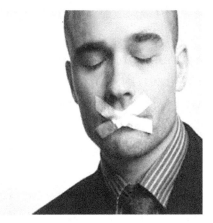

Much of modern-day stress is caused by over-stimulation. If you're like most people, you've got constant noise and distraction happening all around you, and constant demands on your time and attention.

Setting all of that aside for several minutes each day can do <u>WONDERS</u> for your peace of mind and body. Even if you have to wait until late at night or early in the morning to have some quiet time to yourself, <u>do it</u>. Turn off everything that can potentially distract you, like phones, televisions, radios, computers – and just sit and breathe. Let your thoughts flow naturally, but don't latch onto any specific thoughts . . . just let them drift by as you focus on relaxing your body and allowing your mind to rest for a few minutes.

Ideally you should do this for 10-15 minutes a day, but even if you can only escape for a few minutes here and there, it's better than nothing. If you are truly interested in empowering your mind for consistent weight loss, I strongly encourage you to check out my **6-Volume Series, How to Lose Weight & Keep it Off by Transforming the Mind & Behaviors.**

Theater of the Mind

In the next chapter I am going to start directing you to make changes in your diet. That means that you will soon be facing the monsters of hunger and detox symptoms. I wish I could tell you that changing your eating habits and losing fat was 'pain-free', but the truth is that there **IS** some (*temporary*) discomfort involved. But this temporary discomfort is <u>NOTHING</u> in comparison to the amazing fat loss and health benefits that you will gain. Still, here's a meditation that I have used for years to **overcome stress and all of the cravings, hunger and symptoms that come with losing fat and changing eating habits**. Practice it frequently and this entire process will be much smoother... and (yes) easier!

WHITE PAPER (WP) – This mental technique has truly revolutionized my life. It is designed to defuse the endless mental chatter that characterizes the daily lives of many. **(WP)** is easy and simple to implement, yet its effects can be profound.

Here's how it works: From now on, concentrate on slowing down the mind. Spend as much time as possible staring at a piece of *"white paper"* on the movie screen of your mind. Any time you notice that your mind starts to run out of control (*as it so often does*) ... **STOP** and <u>visualize a white piece of paper</u>. I also like to *"see"* myself in a large, empty movie theatre; sitting in a comfortable sofa staring at a **completely blank, bright white screen**.

I sit there in silence waiting for the movie to begin. But the screen <u>ALWAYS </u>stays blank, white and bright. Some days I find myself going to **(WP)** only once or twice. Those are the good days. Then there are days when I'm feeling stressed and vulnerable. Those days, I <u>LIVE</u> in the *'movie theater.'* I'm sure that many times I would have succumbed to stress, junk food and other bad habits if I had not practiced **(WP)**. To me, sitting on that chair at that mental movie theater represents stillness, inner strength, wisdom and discernment. **(WP)** is my own private hideaway where nothing can touch or disturb me. It is the door that leads to the spirit world where I can receive what I lack at that moment.

*Look around you. Masses of people running hectically from one place to another ... their minds constantly processing endless information. But the data is often bad. Most of the "*thoughts*" are tainted with fear, anxiety and all types of emotional anguish. It is no wonder that mental illness continues to increase in today's society! "If so many have not learned to control their own minds and bodies, how then can they live in harmony with their fellows?" Any kind of weight loss regimen exposes our vulnerabilities.

The physical and emotional side-effects of calorie restriction will expose negative thinking patterns. Instead of *"medicating"* your feelings with food, you will be forced to <u>face them head on</u>. Learning to manage these mental juggernauts (*without unhealthy crutches*) is a sure way to achieve ALL of your weight loss goals.

This process is uncomfortable and often painful. But it is worth it. It is the pathway to a happy and healthier life. It absolutely, positively works! So, the best weapon to be successful in losing weight and belly fat is to (*learn*) to <u>keep the mind as blank as possible</u>. God gave us brains to use and by all means productive thought is good.

But <u>endless chatter</u> that offers nothing but fear, anxiety and endless invitations to eat this or that, to forget about weight loss and give up... all of that mental garbage is best discarded through the constant practice of **(WP)**.

What is troubling you? *Is it the job? (*"I just want to quit!"*) *Is there someone that is irking you? (*"I want to put my hands around their neck!"*) *Are hunger pains hitting you hard? (*"Forget all this belly fat crap... I want to eat! Give me a dozen donuts!"*) *Is it the detox symptoms? (**"The heck with the headaches, dizziness and weakness ... give me a cheeseburger!**)

Is it just being alive? ("I don't want to be bothered with anything or anybody! I just want what I want when I want it! Pass the pizza!"*) Whatever the source of discomfort is, take it to **(WP)**. Return to WP when needed throughout this process to keep the mind quiet.

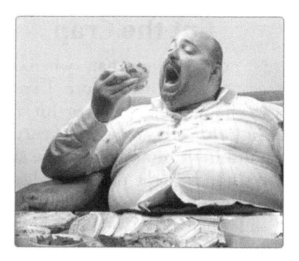

"If what you eat is junk, then that spare roll around your midsection won't budge. What this means is that you have to *cut the crap.*"

Chapter 8
Cut the Crap

There's no question that, when we are stressed, we tend to eat more. I know that hunger and cravings **always hit me the hardest when I am going through a tough moment or am otherwise stressed out**. It's almost as if there is a little food monster inside of me that '*knows*' exactly how and when to hit me with temptation and negativity. When I am centered and feeling good, it hardly ever bothers me. But when I am vulnerable, it comes out from its little hole, guns blazing... bombarding me with all sorts of negativity and temptations.

Handling those moments 'without' giving in is of supreme important if you want to lose belly fat. So I implore you to take these chapters on the '*mind*' seriously and don't just toss them aside. Still, one can have tremendous mental ability and spend eternity in the '*mental movie theater.*' You can be an enlightened Yogi able to keep the mind totally still at all times.

However, **GARBAGE IN, GARBAGE OUT**. If what you eat is junk, then that spare roll around your midsection won't budge. What this means is that you have to *'cut the crap.'* You have to put a lid on poor eating habits. There is <u>no way</u> that you can expect to achieve <u>lasting</u> belly fat loss if you aren't prepared to <u>change the way that you eat</u>.

Willingness and commitment to change is imperative.

How are you doing in that area? Are you willing to do <u>whatever it takes</u> to burn the blubber once and for all? I am going to assume that, since you are reading this book, you **<u>DO</u>** have a level of willingness.

You don't need to have a willpower of steel to get results. Just crack the door open and allow yourself to understand that losing the belly fat is **<u>ABSOLUTELY INDISPENSIBLE</u>** for your long-term health and wellbeing. Can you see that? If you can, then we can use that willingness to move forward. If you are resisting, then I suggest you go back to the beginning and re-read the initial chapters. From this point forward you will be required to let go of the junk. There's no way I want you to finish reading this book and then go and order a pizza or some other trash. I want the message to sink into your psyche loud and clear. Otherwise, belly fat may continue to coat your body for years to come. That isn't what you want, right? How would it feel five years from now if you did nothing and continued to have a (bigger) spare tire? If you can honestly capture the pain of such a scenario, then you know that taking action **NOW** is the only way to avoid it.

Garbage Food

To start seeing belly fat loss right away, we need to **cut the crap from your diet immediately**. If you are anything like I was, then it is possible that your diet is packed with foods very high in fat, sodium and refined sugar. Packaged or canned foods filled with sodium and preservatives that nobody can pronounce. Or perhaps you are a vegan and eat very clean foods, but you eat them in excess. Too much of a good thing can also cause belly fat to accumulate.

The facts are: You want to lose the blubber. What you are doing right now

isn't totally working.

We need to make some changes.   Unless you are shopping at an organic health food market, most of the processed, packaged foods you can buy today are <u>high in calories</u> and loaded with sugar, starch, fat and sodium. These foods do not give your body the nutrition that it needs. Instead, they are like a bomb, raising your blood pressure, cholesterol, and blood sugar levels... not to mention feeding and expanding the belly fat. Foods with a lot of sodium incite water retention which results in that terrible *'bloated'* look that I had for so many years. All of those unnatural, chemical-laden foods need to be eliminated.

They do nothing but increase belly fat and threaten your health.

"Fast food" was the hardest for me to give up because I am lazy and don't like to cook. And once *'online-ordering'* became available, I was hooked. But it is very important to **go through whatever discomfort we need to go through to overcome this trap.** Most fast food is <u>absolute trash</u>. Cheeseburgers, fried chicken, tacos and burritos, pizza and

many Chinese food dishes are super-high in calories and are packed with sugar, fat, MSG and who knows what else. Just <u>ONE</u> meal from these joints gives you massive calories with little or no nutrition. How I managed to survive after tossing that filth into my body for more than 20 years... **I have no idea**. If you want to lose belly fat <u>FOR GOOD</u>, then you <u>MUST</u> become willing to let go of these foods - **starting immediately**. For guidance, here is a list of foods that I want you to cut out right away. Yes, I mean <u>**NOW**</u>. From now on, eat this trash no more. You'll see the belly fat start to melt off like you wouldn't believe.

Banned Foods List:

*****Salt** - You don't need added salt. It bloats you and feeds the belly fat.

* **Sugar** - Belly fat's best friend and your worst enemy. Steer clear. Some fruit during the day is fine. No more.

* **Fried Foods:** This is junk and will only make you fatter. Cut it out for good!

* **Cheese** - Soy Cheese is Ok on Occasion

* **Dairy Products** - Drink only fat-free milk

* **Red Meat** - only lean fish, turkey or chicken. No more than 4 oz. per serving

* **Alcohol** - One cup of wine daily is fine. Alcohol has a LOT of calories and feeds the belly fat

* **Butter or Margarine** - This is a biggie. Has a lot of fat that goes directly to the belly. Cut it out completely.

* **Fruit Juices** - Packed with 'natural' sugar, but sugar nonetheless. <u>ONE</u> 6oz glass in the AM would be fine. No more.

* **Regular Ketchup** (except low sodium) -

***Soda and Junk Food of ANY Kind**. Pizza, cheeseburgers, pastries, donuts, fried foods... fast food of ANY kind is OUT unless it's a salad. And in that case, skip the dressing. Use a small sprinkle of olive oil and balsamic vinegar instead.

Keep it Simple

Believe it or not, eating healthy <u>does not</u> have to become a trail of tears or something extremely difficult to achieve. Neither does it necessarily have to be super expensive. Yes, one could easily spend a lot more money in the market shopping for healthy foods. But there are cost-effective options within your reach. Need *'fast food'*? How about fruits and vegetables?

How about buying a juicer and **starting to juice fruits and veggies regularly and replace a meal**? What I love about fruits and veggies is that most of them can be eaten raw.

Steaming vegetables like broccoli, cauliflower and carrots takes only like ten minutes and is very satisfying. Add a lean piece of fish or chicken (*no more than eight ounces per serving*) and a baked potato, and you've got a very nice (*and clean*) meal.

If you are able, my recommendation is that you buy organic fruits and veggies. I read an article recently about all of the pesticides that are sprayed on produce these days to make them big and keep them fresh. I was horrified.

Definitely go organic if you are able. If not, then you have to scrub the produce thoroughly under warm water **BEFORE** you cook and eat it.

Fat-Burning Formula

Let's do a quick recap here and see what you can start to do to lose belly fat immediately:

*Cut the crap in the banned foods list

*Increase your daily intake of fruits and vegetables

*Drink at least one gallon of water daily (more about this shortly)

*Work at lowering stress levels in your daily life

Want to supercharge fat loss? ->Start exercising at least three times weekly for 30 minutes. Like I said, start at the beginning and do what you can. **But do it.**

If you take these steps <u>ONLY</u>, you will start to see <u>very noticeable</u> belly fat loss within two weeks or less. There's no reason why you can't lose as much as two inches of flab every month. You will be surprised. Losing belly fat may seem like a daunting, very difficult task... but it really isn't.

Yes, there is initial discomfort *(hunger &*

detox symptoms) while the body breaks its addiction to junk foods and/or overeating, but this uncomfortable process doesn't last very long. And the feeling of wellness and freedom that you will gain is tremendous.

Try to make the basis of your diet **75% or more** all-natural, whole foods, just like they come from nature. That means lean protein from poultry, fish, beef, pork, and beans and legumes; plenty of fruit and vegetables in their natural forms; whole grains rather than refined white bread, pasta and rice; and healthy fats like olive oil and avocadoes. If you eat a lot of dairy products like milk, cheese and yogurt, you may want to opt for versions that are lower in saturated fat, or even soy versions if your digestive system doesn't tolerate dairy products well.

Eating processed foods occasionally shouldn't cause a problem for most people, but you definitely don't want to make them the main part of your daily diet. You may find like many other people have that just improving the quality of the food you eat by reducing chemicals, sodium, sugar and fat has a dramatic, slimming effect on your stomach as well as the rest of your body.

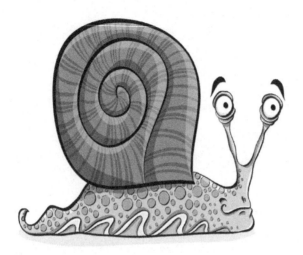

"Another cause of belly fat is a sluggish metabolism. When your metabolism isn't functioning efficiently, you are more likely to store fat."

Chapter 9
Slow Metabolism

Another key cause of belly fat accumulation is a slow metabolism. If you have not gone to get full blood work recently, I encourage you to do so. If you have been having a hard time losing weight, it is possible you might have an <u>underactive thyroid</u>. Such was the case with me. The condition is called **hypothyroidism**. When this illness is present, even your most honest and aggressive attempts to lose belly fat can fall short.

The flips side is **hyperthyroidism**, which means that the thyroid gland is *'overactive'* and the person is unable to <u>GAIN</u> weight. My precious uncle has struggled with this condition. He has always been <u>very</u> thin. At first I envied him and wished he could pass on to me some of that *'hyper'* stuff. But as he has gotten older, he has lost more and more weight and his health has been threatened. Both hyper and hypothyroidism are dangerous conditions and need to be treated ASAP. The good news is that, in many cases, learning how to eat and getting active (*as described in the previous chapter*) could help one improve (*and even eliminate*) the condition. That's what happened to me. But please do get blood tests done if you haven't done so recently. It can help identify hidden conditions and anything else that could be affecting your health and limiting your weight loss results.

Eat Six Times Daily

The **ONE** step that helped me <u>the most</u> to accelerate my metabolism was simply this: **Going from three to six meals per day.** This meal structure includes breakfast, mid-morning snack, lunch, mid-afternoon snack, dinner and evening snack. The metabolism is like a fire. Let me give you an analogy to illustrate.

Imagine that you were stranded in a very cold place and needed to keep a fire burning to survive the night. Would you be better off dumping a huge amount of firewood at once, or would the fire burn longer and keep you warmer if you added small amounts of wood frequently? Of course, the answer is the latter.

The more frequently you eat (*observing the banned foods list*), the better you will feel and the more energy you will have. Consequently, the metabolism will work evenly and continuously, which results in faster fat loss. Having larger meals with less frequency is like dumping a large amount of wood into the fire.

You will get one heck of blaze initially, but it will die out sooner and not provide as much heat (energy) as it would if you added wood more sparingly.

This is what causes the monster cravings that keep people trapped in binging and overeating for years. If you want to disconnect the cravings and speed up the fat loss process, eat more frequently.

The six-meals-per-day structure helped me to lose the last 30 pounds of belly fat that I was struggling with, and it has helped me to keep all the weight that I lost off for 12 years now.

To help you see how this works, here is a sample menu from a typical day in my life:

Sample Menu

Breakfast 8:00 AM

1 Cup of Oatmeal with 1 Cup Skim Milk, a Handful of Raisins or Plums

Three Egg Whites mixed with, 3 OZ Ground Turkey

1 Cup of Green Tea with Stevia

Mid-Morning Snack 10AM

1 Apple or Pear Mixed With One Cup of Nonfat Yogurt (Plain)

OR, **ONE** Apple, Pear, Banana or Other Fruit

Lunch - Noon

Big salad with lettuce, tomato and other veggies you may like. For dressing, use olive oil (no more than 1 teaspoon) and balsamic vinegar.

1 Envelope of Low-Sodium Tuna

1 4OZ Baked Potato or Sweet Potato

Mid-Afternoon Snack 3PM

Same as before - I usually have a piece of fruit mixed with yogurt. At this time in the afternoon, I also drink another cup of green tea. Green tea has energy-boosting and body-heating properties. It will help to give you a pep as well as calm hunger pangs. In addition to green tea, seltzer water (sparkling water/club soda) is great to navigate hunger.

Dinner - 6PM

Six-to-eight ounces of chicken, fish or ground turkey (I like to make turkey patties)

Large salad as the one eaten for lunch

Steamed Broccoli, Cauliflower and Carrots (most supermarkets have prepackaged vegetable combinations that are ready to steam and eat).

4OZ Baked Potato or Sweet Potato **OR** 4OZ of Whole Wheat or Whole Grain Pasta **OR** 4 OZ of Brown Rice

Evening Snack - 8PM

Big salad with 3OZ Chicken, Fish or Ground Turkey - No carbohydrates.

A piece of fruit with Non-fat Yogurt

Cup of Chamomile Tea - Chamomile tea is

great to drink at night because it will help soothe hunger as well as calm you and get you ready for bed.

You should not eat anything at least two hours prior to turning in. Sometimes I also take one 500 mg tablet of Tryptophan at night to help me sleep. Tryptophan is an awesome amino acid that helps to stabilize mood.

At this point I'm done eating for the day and drink only water until 8AM the following morning.

Again -> NEVER EAT FOR THE LAST TWO HOURS BEFORE YOU GO TO BED. Do you ingest a large portion of your daily calories a few hours before bedtime?

When your body is at rest, all of your metabolic processes slow down so you don't burn as many calories as you would during the day while you are actively moving around.

When you eat large portions of food shortly before you go to bed, many of those calories are going to be stored as fat. Unfortunately, some people eat very few calories all day long, then gulp down a large dinner – and then munch on snacks all evening before they go to bed! Throughout the day they may have ingested 500 to 700 calories, and then 2,000 to 3,000 calories right before they go to bed. Bad idea! Tape your mouth shut if you have to. But eat no more!

12-Hour Daily Fasting

As you can see by the sample menu, this is not about starving, but rather about <u>eating smart</u>. That is a whole lot of food to eat in one day. **But it is clean food eaten frequently.** The metabolism will kick into high gear and help you to lose fat faster. In addition, you will be fasting 12 hours daily from 8PM to 8AM.

Twelve hours of daily nighttime fasting gives the body time to digest the food as well as perform some very important housekeeping duties such as detoxification, fat burning, healing and tissue repair. If everyone gave the body at least 12 hours daily of fasting, a lot of obesity and disease would be wiped out. This nightly period of **<u>NOT</u>** eating is extremely important and beneficial. So once you have eaten your last meal of the day... shut your trap!

No more food until breakfast!

At first it may be rough and you may be hungry within an hour after you eat the last meal. The hunger may harass you all night long. Get up and drink water. Go back to bed. Don't eat! Trust me, you will feel light and very nice in the morning. And, after a few weeks of daily nighttime fasting, the hunger will go away and you'll do fine.

You will sleep better, longer and wake up refreshed. If you add this six-meal/nightly fasting structure to all of the other steps we've already discussed, there is **ZERO** reason why you cannot lose **ALL** of the belly fat. It has worked wonders for me and I was the worst of the worst as far as obesity and poor eating. Now it is YOUR time to make it happen!

Chapter 10
Increase Water Intake

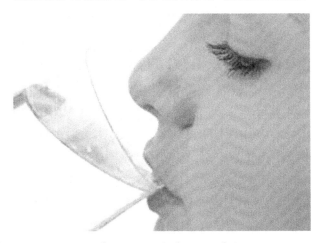

If you want to lose weight and improve your health and life - then a good way to start is by curtailing the intake of caffeine, sodas and artificially-flavored drinks. Whether or not you are fasting, drinking more water daily **MUST** be incorporated into your lifestyle.

INCREASE YOUR WATER INTAKE.

Doesn't sound like much, does it? Well, **IT'S A LOT!** Just starting to drink more water each day helps the body to flush out disease-causing toxins and pungent fecal matter adhered to the walls of the colon.

The water can notably soothe gastrointestinal conditions as constipation and irritable bowel syndrome, which are often interrelated and run rampant in the US.

HERE'S THE BOTTOM LINE: Drink one half-gallon of water <u>every day for the rest of your life</u>... period. And, guess what? Doing this consistently, water studies indicate, can foster gradual weight loss **WITHOUT** exercise or special diets. Sounds too good to be true... what's the catch? Well, there really is no catch. The concept is that cool water forces the body to burn roughly 60 calories more per day because it has to <u>WARM</u> the water up to its system-wide temperature.

It isn't much of a shock that most of us <u>DO NOT</u> drink sufficient water. I talk to people all the time that tell me they simply do not like the taste of water; others simply are unwilling to do it. Many are addicted to caffeine and/or sugar-infested juices and soft-drinks. Any time they feel thirst, the farthest thing on their minds is to drink water. In fact, they will drink any beverage under God's blessed sun - <u>EXCEPT</u> water.

Their bodily functions are somewhat impaired, making all of the organs and muscles work much harder than they should. If you fall into any of these categories, then hopefully I can motivate you to start drinking more water.

The message I want to bring to you is very simple: **DRINK MORE WATER!** The benefits you can gain are tremendous when you do it <u>daily and consistently</u>. If you are interested in improving your health and losing weight, then this is a simple action you can take <u>TODAY</u> to start moving towards your health-related goals. In order to burn fat efficiently your organs need to be functioning properly, and for that to happen your body needs to be fully hydrated. Need I say more?

Chapter 11
Portion Control

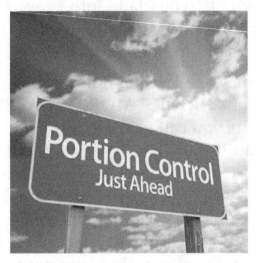

The truth is that most of us have gained belly fat because we eat too much. We nibble, graze and overeat. You can follow the healthiest diet in the world. However, if you overeat, then the belly fat will continue to haunt you. I know many people who have eaten very clean diets their whole lives. Yet they are overweight because they don't control their portions.

Here's the key: Every time that you eat, make it a point to come away satisfied but still *'a little bit'* hungry. There is <u>NO </u>reason why you should be stuffed after any meal. If you are stuffed, then you ate too much and are going in the wrong direction. Only <u>YOU</u> know how much you eat and what quantities you consume.

Start reducing the portions that you serve on your plate.

Cut them by 1/4... do that for a few weeks, and then practice cutting it by 1/2. I say '*practice*' because this is about progress, not perfection. If you stumble, try again on the next meal. But keep going! Keep trying!

Continue until you are able to eat <u>HALF</u> of the food that you used to eat. If you do that, your belly fat problem will end and your life and health will be transformed.

It has been proven that **the less we eat, the healthier we will likely be and the longer we will likely live**. Not even the most delicious, mouth-watering meal can compare to the feeling I have when I wake up in the morning feeling light, clear and refreshed. Formerly, I would wake up feeling like a truck had run over me because I had stuffed myself with food the previous day. Therefore, rather than work on detoxification, healing and tissue repair, the body had to *'stay up all night'* digesting all of the crap that I had eaten. I robbed myself of the restorative power of a good night's sleep - all to please my belly. Trust me, eating less will not only help you to burn the belly fat faster, but you will begin to feel a lot better physically, emotionally... every which way.

As I said, the key is to **walk away from each meal feeling just a little hungry**. Get used to being a little hungry all of the time. There is this notion that hunger needs to be appeased at all times and without question.

Why? That is **NOT** the lifestyle that is conducive to lasting fat loss and health. We **MUST** learn to master our appetite, and the best way to accomplish that is by starting **TODAY** to practice portion control. Did you know that the average person's stomach can hold about a quart? That's about 4 cups worth of food and liquid. The problem is that it's possible to stretch the stomach to accommodate more than that – and boy do some of us push the limits! Over time, you can stretch your stomach so much that normal portion sizes are no longer enough to satisfy you. If you were to poll a bunch of people with naturally flat stomachs, you'd probably find that most of them are <u>light eaters</u>. Even if they can put away a fair amount of calories in a day, they probably eat only small amounts of food each time they eat.

For example, they'll have just half a sandwich instead of a whole one (**or two**). They'll have "*just a sliver*" of cake instead of a big chunk. They "*peck*" at food just like birds peck at feed on the ground, **eating little bits here and there but never overeating a lot of food at one time**.

Regardless of the size of your body or whether you have belly fat or not, **eating smaller portions of food can only benefit you!** It helps you avoid taxing your digestive system any more than necessary, which leaves more energy and vitality for the rest of your body. You can even take this method to the next level by deciding to eat **<u>ONLY</u>** when you are physically hungry, and then only eating as much as it takes to satisfy your hunger, <u>but no more than that</u>.

If you already do this you may be wondering, *"doesn't everyone eat this way"*? No. Many people develop the habit of eating for every other reason <u>except</u> for physical hunger, and then keep right on eating way past the point of satiety.

If this describes you, start today by listening to your body's hunger signals, and then stop eating as soon as you no longer feel hungry (*but you aren't yet really "full" either*). You may be pleasantly surprised by how little food it takes to satisfy you, and the increase in energy you get from not taxing your system with too much food – **not to mention the almost immediate shrinking of your belly and other overweight areas!**

Chapter 12
Limit Alcohol Consumption

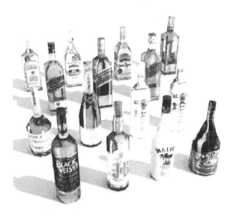

Alcohol has a huge amount of empty calories. When I say empty, I mean that they provide no nutritional value. Too much alcohol consumption is one of the biggest causes of belly fat. I'm sure you've heard the term *'beer belly.'* It isn't a figure of speech; it's an unfortunate side effect of too much drinking. Let me say it again:

Alcohol has a lot of calories.

If you have just a drink occasionally and budget the calories into your daily caloric intake, it's probably not going to cause too many problems. But if you routinely go out and have one, two, three or more drinks, then all of those excess calories will go directly to the belly. Unless you are doing three hours daily or cardio, it simply isn't possible for the body to burn off all of those calories. Even worse, alcohol lowers inhibitions.

You may find yourself in a social function, a bit 'tipsy' and surrounded by food. You will be vulnerable and could end up overeating. That happened to me many times and I would always wake up feeling terrible, full of guilt, frustration and totally demoralized.

You can do a great job with your diet for weeks and totally throw a wrench into the process with just one night of too much alcohol.

And, if you end up giving in to food as well, you won't be very happy at all the next morning. And when we get frustrated like this, we are much more open to fall prey to the *screw it* syndrome I talked about earlier.

Moderation is Key

12 oz. beer, regular	140 calories
12 oz. beer, light	100 calories
1.5 oz. hard liquor	80 calories
5 oz. wine	130 calories
12 oz. wine cooler	200 calories
4 oz. liqueur	130 calories

Look, I am not saying that you have to become a teetotaler. One cup of wine daily is fine. If you're a beer drinker, do not have more than two or three a week - even if it is the 'light' kind. Hard booze like gin, rum, whiskey and tequila should be avoided altogether.

Sweet liqueurs like brandy and cognac are packed with sugar and are banned. If you are in the habit of drinking several times a week, or even daily, do what you can to cut down as much as possible.

That doesn't mean you can't go out with

your friends and have a good time, but you can easily drink seltzer water with lime instead of beer. Or have just one drink and then switch to water. Before attending any social functions, be sure to eat something light and nutritious like a salad or some lean protein so you aren't hungry. You'll be less tempted to overindulge on sweet or fatty foods.

Chapter 13
Hormones

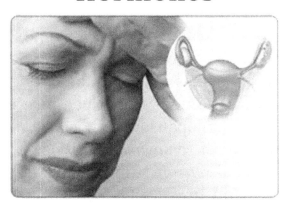

Whether you are male or female, hormonal changes will inevitably happen which can contribute to increases in belly fat. Most people become less active as they age. This causes the metabolism to slow down which, in turn, results in faster weight gain - mostly in belly fat. And hormones play a key role in these age-related changes. Being aware of them and, more importantly, starting to take action NOW is imperative if you wish to lose the belly fat and safeguard your health.

Women: Menopause

Menopause is recognized as a factor that

contributes to the accumulation of belly fat. If you are going through menopause, then it is probable that you have begun to see some changes in your body's shape. The majority of women will gain 15-20 pounds during menopause. Most of the weight gain, however, comes slowly - about <u>one pound per year</u>. Women who experience early or surgical menopause (*menopause resulting from surgical removal of both of the ovaries for medical reasons*) may gain weight more rapidly and drastically. You'll likely notice that weight distribution throughout your body is not as even as it used to be.

To be sure, maintaining weight during menopause is challenging because hormonal fluctuations directly impact appetite, metabolism, and fat storage. Some women do put on excessive weight during menopause (*more than 20 pounds*). This could be a symptom that there is a more serious issue with your hormone levels. So if you find yourself gaining an inordinate amount of weight, please see your doctor right away. Hormone replacement therapy is one treatment option that you may want to discuss with your doctor. There are some studies which indicate that replacement therapy can reduce the body's tendency to store more fat during menopause. Still, the treatment is not without its risks. Some of the risks associated with hormone replacement therapy are blood clots, stroke, heart disease and breast cancer. You want to make sure that the 'cure' isn't worse than the condition itself. So please tread very carefully and **<u>NEVER</u>** jump into any treatment without first discussing it thoroughly with a qualified health care professional.

Men: Low Testosterone

This is a condition that I myself have had to deal with, so I know just how frustrating it can be. Testosterone is the main male hormone produced in the testicles. It develops a male's distinctiveness such as height, voice tone and facial/pubic hair, among others. Testosterone controls bone and muscle mass, sperm production and sex drive. The female body (*adrenal gland and ovaries*) also produces this hormone, albeit in much smaller amounts. There are plenty of studies out there indicating that low testosterone may be connected to weight gain. I am certain that such was my case.

One particular study I found interesting was carried out in 2006 of 2,000 men 45+ years of age. It showed that **obese males were more than two times apt to have low levels of testosterone than those who maintained a healthy body weight**. That was quite the eye-opener for me. Other studies have shown that testosterone levels fall in the measure that **Body Mass Index** rises.

In other words, the fatter we get, the more testosterone levels fall. There are additional studies which link low testosterone to a surge in body fat, especially in the belly. And this can cause a myriad of health problems, including fatigue, loss of interest in life, reduced sex drive and mood swings, as well as heart disease, high blood pressure and the dreaded Type II diabetes.

None of the studies seem to be 100% conclusive, but the writing is definitely on the wall. There is the option of testosterone replacement therapy. There are studies that have shown that testosterone replacement therapy has helped to lower triglycerides, blood glucose levels and... fat storage. But deciding to take part in this form of treatment is something that needs to be discussed with your doctor as it does have its risks. I personally chose not to take part in testosterone replacement therapy. Instead, I have had good results with a natural supplement called *TribuPlex 750*. I am simply sharing this information with you, not prescribing or telling you to take the supplement. You can look into it and decide if it may be for you.

So what can one do to traverse all of these hormonal challenges without blowing up like a balloon? Well, the answer is as simple as following **ALL** of the suggestions that we have looked at thus far. Don't worry, I will list them all at the end when we wrap up. But I think you can see that we need to hit this belly fat issue from all angles.

Half measures will produce little or nothing.

Whether you are male or female, there are simply too many health risks related to excess belly fat. But you don't need to be dismayed. There is hope. Even if you are very overweight, taking assertive action can start to reverse a lot of the damage. That way, hormones can be managed more effectively without resulting in massive weight gain. Rather than just accepting excess weight as an inevitable part of growing older, roll up your sleeves and get to work! There are plenty of extremely active, fit and healthy people that are middle-aged and beyond. You can be one too.

Chapter 14
Genetics

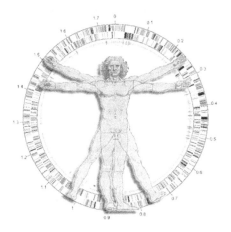

Another reason why many people are overweight is because of family genetics. Take a moment to think about your immediate family members. Do your parents, siblings and grandparents have excess fat around their middles? If most or many of them do, it's possible that you have a genetic disposition to belly fat.

People with this disposition are often referred to as having an "apple" shape to their bodies, meaning they tend to accumulate fat around the middle but not so much elsewhere. Compare this to a person with a *"pear"* shape, accumulating more fat in the buttocks and thighs rather than the stomach. However, even if you have a genetic disposition, it doesn't mean you are doomed to have an accumulation of belly fat forever.

It is important for you to learn to separate yourself from your family and start to make different decisions for your own life. Just because Uncle Bob is fat, that doesn't mean that you also have to be.

If that was the case, then I should still be obese because my grandfather was... and so on. Even though genetics always play a role, it is our **PERSONAL DECISIONS AND BEHAVIORS** which will eventually tell the final tale.

Decide right now that you're going to set aside excuses and do whatever you can to change your diet and exercise habits and take control of your own health and well-being.

Keep in mind that it's not just genes that are passed down through the generations, but **<u>HABITS</u>** are too. You may have learned some unhealthy habits from your relatives, but <u>you have the power to change</u> those, which will make your results different from theirs. You may have to take a tough stand at first because, if you have a close family, some of them may resist and even resent your efforts to eat and behave differently.

Genetics are very powerful and can literally pull you in and keep you locked into counterproductive habits for a lifetime.

Don't allow it. <u>Stand your ground</u>... the family will come around eventually. And you will be a powerful force of change that everyone can look up to. Not only that, but **you will be passing on a whole new inheritance to your children**, one of personal responsibility, health and freedom.

You can literally break chains that have held your family for generations **<u>IF</u>** you are willing to do the work.

To do this, it is crucial to become aware of the inner world of thoughts that lies behind the surface, constantly speaking to you and asking you to reinforce the negative.

The Inner Voice

One of the most powerful tools that I discovered to help me lose weight and keep it off was to <u>identify the voices inside of me that wanted to sabotage my progress</u>. These 'voices' are made up of an internal conversation such as:

"What's the use, you might as well stop now because you'll never make it. Oh, this is a waste of time. You are too weak. You don't have what it takes. You're a loser. You're ugly and flat and nobody wants you (this one was very strong with me). This isn't worth the effort. I'd rather be eating... resting... Sleeping... watching TV etc..."

I realized that right before I did something foolish (*like break my diet, eat junk food, skip a workout and so on*) there was **a conversation within talking me into doing so**. I believe that these behaviors and belief systems are part of that genetic predisposition, so it is <u>imperative to learn to identify them</u>.

Take some time and see if you can identify the voices and conversations in your mind that sabotage your weight loss. Write them down. Next time you are presented with those negative voices, you will have the option to give in (*again*) **OR** to reject them. If you can understand that '*giving in*' will only produce more and more failure, then your <u>**ONLY**</u> option becomes to challenge them.

Not to do so would be the worst form of self-betrayal because you would be feeding into thought patterns that <u>YOU KNOW</u> are leading you astray. It is like knowing that somebody means you harm but ignoring that fact and going along with them anyways.

Would you do that? I don't think so. It may not be easy at first to say <u>**NO**</u>... but you <u>**MUST**</u> if you want to find lasting victory. Not only is it important to say <u>**NO**</u>, but it is also essential to **act in direct opposition to what the voices/thoughts are suggesting**. If the suggestion is that you skip the workout, say <u>**NO**</u> and go anyways - <u>even if you have to drag your elbows on the</u>

<u>ground</u>. If the invitation is to stop at a donut shop, say **<u>NO</u>** and drive by it without stopping. If the thought is that you are weak and that you will never make it, say **<u>NO</u>** and continue to follow your fat loss program.

The more you stand your ground and say NO, the weaker the voices will become until, eventually, they will be just a minor irritation.

And that internal work will manifest powerfully on the outside because, rather than giving in, you will be reinforcing your new, healthy habits. And that reinforcement, over time, will wipe out the belly fat because the internal opposition will have been destroyed. A lot of people fail to pay attention to this internal dynamic and focus only on the externals. When they fall short of their goals, they fill themselves with remorse and self-hatred, not realizing that in doing so they are continuing to reinforce the very foe that is holding them back.

Chapter 15
Mastering Food

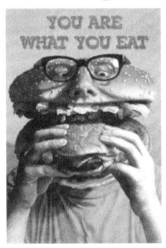

It's all about what we eat, really. Eating poorly (or too much) is what causes body fat to surge the fastest. The point we always emphasize is this; permanent weight loss and health are best attained when one is constantly learning about the food one eats, what it contains, and how it positively or negatively is affecting our minds and bodies.

I swam in a pool of ignorance for years; eating whatever and whenever without any clue as to what food was, and how it could help enhance or destroy life. Truly, the picture above is a very good depiction of what I was rapidly becoming through my obesity, binging and overeating. So let us join together in this quest for understanding and, eventually, mastering food. To master food is to master our bodies. And to master our bodies is to master our minds and emotions.

To master our minds and emotions is to master our lives. Believe it or not, your body detox and weight loss quest has existential significance. If you stick to it and resist the urge to return to old habits, I can tell you that the physical and mental breakthroughs that await you are beyond imagination. Food is the source of power - it is up to you to learn how to use it in your favor, rather than as an agent of self-annihilation.

You Are What You Eat

The old adage "**You are What you Eat**," is true. Food can be toxic. The junk food that so many eat in high quantities (*soda, burgers, French fries, pizza, candy etc.*) is full of all types of destructive elements that cut many lives short. You probably have heard of many of them, including chemicals, free radicals, as well as excessive amounts of sugar and Trans fats. These foods, as we all know, are very high in calories and have little or no nutritional value. Worse yet, for many people - especially in the US - this type of poisonous food represents the bulk of their daily diets. It is little wonder that the obesity epidemic is spiraling out of control.

Understanding Food

The weight loss and fitness we seek is attained by eating less, of course. But more importantly it is about **eating right**. You can be the most active person in the universe.

However, if you do not take hold of your eating habits, the benefits will be paltry and you will find yourself constantly returning to substandard health. I want you to use food to your advantage rather than to your detriment.

One of the most constructive ways you can start using food to your advantage is to **learn how to scrutinize and understand food labels**. This may sound silly, but I have learned that 90 percent of people hardly ever - or never - read labels. Or perhaps they misread the label, which can be even worse.

In the US, the **Food and Drug Administration** requires that anything in a container (*and almost anything edible you buy*) has to have a label with nutritional facts, including serving size, servings per container, calories, fat, carbohydrates and proteins. We have all seen them, right?

Many labels also have in-depth information as to how much sugar and/or salt the particular food contains. I am shocked by the obscene amount of sodium (*salt*) in most canned and frozen foods. This is the case with even so called "diet" or "low fat" selections. When I started to actually read and understand labels, I found that almost 100 percent of what I was eating was toxic and damaging to my body.

Serving Sizes

Please be aware that if the label says that it has "*two servings per container,*" then all the nutritional information in the label of that particular product needs to be doubled. I am sure that you probably know this already, but I think it was worth mentioning for the sake of what we are discussing. A large container of frozen food may say, for example, "four servings in a box." If you eat the whole box, you are eating four times the amount of fat or calories in the label. In this case the *"serving size"* would be one-fourth of that particular box, not the entire box as many people often believe.

Bottom line: Make sure you check both *Serving Size and Servings per Container.* Nine times out of ten the servings per container exceed the serving size, meaning that if you consume that entire product, then the fat, calories, carbohydrates (etc.) have to be multiplied times the servings per container.

Chapter 16
More on Sugar, Fat & Starches

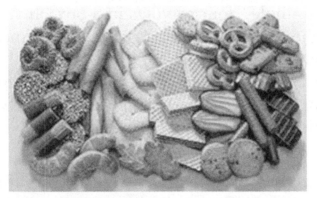

I am horrified by the abuse of fat, sugar and starches and how this practice is literally making millions sick and sending them to an early grave. When you combine this with chronic inactivity, the result undoubtedly is obesity and sickness.

It is my aim to give you a message that goes **BEYOND BELLY FAT** so that you can permanently attain a leaner and healthier you. Perhaps starch and inactivity have been a trap for you. Don't worry. There is a way out. Here we are going to get slightly technical in regards to white starches and sugars and how they negatively affect your body. We also will provide suggestions you can use to get your back on track and help you achieve your weight loss and fitness goals. But as with everything, this is a process. Be good to yourself and remember: *the tortoise won the race.* Make slow but steady changes and you will definitely reap the results. **CONTINUE** to take action until you develop new eating and lifestyle habits that support and enhance YOUR fat loss and health improvement efforts.

Starch Sabotage

The other thing you can do is to take a food inventory and remove as much refined starches and sugars from your diet as you can. Do it for good! In the US, there are more stomach diseases than in any other country in the world. The reason? Abuse of starches and sugars - to a great extent. In Asian countries, for the most part, they do not have problems with obesity or the barrage of gastrointestinal illnesses we see in the West.

Stomach cancer, diverticulitis, colitis - all of these diseases are rare. One of my very good friends has been a nurse for more than 30 years and she says she has **NEVER** come across and Asian patient needing a gastric bypass surgery. Maybe one or two have been overweight. Most are lean, she said. She told me that during the 16 days she spent in China some years ago, the only overweight people she saw were in the large cities of Hong Kong and Beijing. Guess what? That is where the fast food restaurants are! Coincidence? I don't think so.

Food Combinations

Thirty years ago, the concept of food combinations came up for the first time. It centers on the premise that, for example, starch and protein should not be eaten together. Refined starches such as bread or potatoes should be eaten with a salad or a vegetable - not meat as it is done customarily.

Why? Because the combination of refined starch and meat often end up becoming an indigestible lump in your stomach. This puts significant strain in your digestive system and fosters the accumulation of belly fat. In the US, the combination of fat and starch represents the main staple of the diet. What is a hamburger? Fat from the meat, starch from the bread. What is pizza? Fat from the cheese, starch from the dough. What is a hot dog? What is a submarine sandwich? Same fat/starch combination with a different disguise.

Escaping the Starch and Fat Trap

What is your diet mostly made up of? How do you combine foods and which are the ones that make up the largest portion of your daily consumption?

For many overweight *(and highly toxic)* people, it is <u>almost certain</u> that **fat and starch are combined in almost every meal**. This is a very harmful practice that, over years, can seriously affect your health and cut your life short. I want you to consider removing all *"white"* starches from your diet or, at the very least, only eat them once a day.

I included these in the banned foods we looked at earlier, but their consumption is do damaging that I thought it was worthwhile to mention it again. Foods like white rice, white bread, enriched pasta, most breakfast cereals, crackers cookies, cakes and chips, should be seriously curtailed or - better yet - **eradicated**. And remember: fasting even once a week can be a very powerful practice toward weight loss and better health. Or, at the least, try skipping one meal every three days. Do what you can. But do it! It works, it really does!

Chapter 17
Inactivity

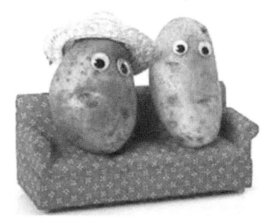

I talked about getting active a little while ago. However, I want to emphasize it again because it is the most indispensable part of your fat loss program.

The weight gain/ weight loss equation remains the same: **Calories In - Calories Burned = Weight Loss or Weight Gain**, depending on the amount of calories consumed.

We all know that the most successful method to belly fat and attain optimum health is to not only decrease calorie intake, but to also increase the amount of calories burned via some sort of exercise. I come from a family of mostly heavy people. The genetic predisposition to obesity has been verified along with many other diseases. But, as we discussed in the chapter on genetics, that does not mean that you should accept being overweight because others in your family are.

That is not true. In fact, my message to you is that you **CAN** make the change! You **CAN** break patterns that perhaps other people in your family were unable to overcome.

Upon pondering this thought, **I realize that it has been increased physical activity which has helped me the most to stay lean and healthy**. I am very strict with my diet and follow a structure very similar to the one I presented earlier.

However, I am not sure if I would have been able to maintain my health and weight if I wasn't active. When, for one reason or another, I become inactive, I feel the pain almost immediately. Overall, I always become restless and uncomfortable when I go more than a week without exercising. The insidious thoughts of eating in excess start to circle around my head like vultures. To me, inactivity is poison. It traps me and causes bad eating habits to reemerge. **And here's the truth:** all living things move - plants, animals, humans.

The only organism that is perfectly still is one that is dead.

Why then do beings created to move (*equipped with muscles, ligaments and bones that support and conduce movement*) by their very purpose and design, lie still for days, weeks, months and years? It does not make sense.

Chapter 18
Action Steps

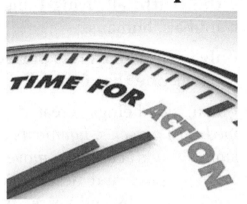

Alright let's now look at all of this material in a list of **action steps** that you can work on from now on:

***Start a journal** where you can write about your fat loss process.

***Get a body fat measurement** and compare it to the chart that we looked at earlier so that you can assess where you stand. Log the results in the journal. What is your body fat percentage?

What is your lean body mass percentage? In which category are you? Healthy? Obese? What is your target body fat percentage?

How many pounds of body fat do you have to lose to reach that goal? Write about why reaching this goal is important to you and what you are willing to do to reach it.

*Effective immediately, work at <u>reducing your levels of stress</u> by putting to practice the suggestions that we talked about in that chapter. Incorporate some time of meditation on your daily schedule. This is not about religion, it is about having a time of total calm and silence. If you do practice a religion, then by all means you can incorporate the meditation into your devotional time.

***Practice the White Paper technique** and get used to visiting the 'mind theater' every time you start to feel overwhelmed. Work at 'not reacting' to the daily annoyances that try to take your peace of mind. Don't allow it. Remember that excessive stress contributes to belly fat storage, not only because we eat more but because of the increased accumulation of cortisol in the body. So stress management is key for long term fat loss.

***Get active:** go through the chapter on this

topic and make up your mind as to what type of activity you are going to start implementing in your life - at least three times weekly. Like I said, start where you are and do not try to run a triathlon the first week. Take it slow, be consistent and you will see the results.

*Cut the Crap: Effective immediately, cut out from your diet all of the junk on the *'banned foods list'*. Increase your daily intake of fruits and vegetables. Follow the six-meals-per day structure even if it is at first uncomfortable. Most of us have had eating habits that are totally unbridled like wild horses in the Wild West. You may resist following an eating structure at first, but eventually it will become a part of your lifestyle and you will be very happy that you did it.

*Practice fasting 12 hours each night, from the time that you eat your last meal, to the time that you have breakfast the following day. As we saw, not eating during this time period gives the body time to focus on detoxification, healing and tissue repair and allows you to rest deeply and wake up refreshed and restored.

*Start to <u>drink at the very least half a gallon of water daily</u>.

*Work at **cutting the portions that you eat, initially by 1/4 and eventually by 1/2.** This is an ongoing assignment. If you are diligent and persistent, you can reduce your food intake by 50% within a year. That will have a huge impact on the loss of belly fat.

* **Limit alcohol intake**

* **Consider hormonal changes** and see your doctor about treatment options and whether they can help you or not.

* **Consider whether genetics is something that has contributed to the belly fat**, and make a commitment to yourself that you will overcome the challenge by making different choices for yourself.

Just because your family is overweight and eats poorly doesn't mean that you, too, have to follow the same path. You can break free and create a whole new inheritance of freedom and personal responsibility, for yourself as well as your children.

*Learn to identify the inner voices that are always beckoning you to give in and cut corners, practice saying **NO** to them and acting in direct opposition to them.

The more you say **NO** and continue to stand your ground, the faster you will see progress on the outside. And that progress will be **PERMANENT** because you will have overcome the destructive voices that led you to behave in unhealthy ways.

*Keep going through these points over and over until you can adopt all of them into your lifestyle. Work at optimizing the implementation of each of these points.

There will always be room for improvement. If you give yourself to the task, within a few weeks you will start to see the belly fat shrink. Within months, the belly fat will be against the ropes... and - if you hang on and are patient - you will find in time that the belly fat problem has been solved.

Chapter 19
Beyond the Blubber

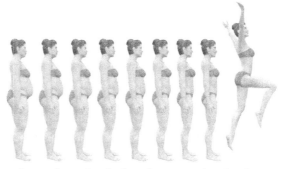

I have bombarded the living daylights out of you. I realize that this is a lot to absorb at once. The thing to keep in mind about belly fat is that it's not **JUST** about the belly. There is no evil belly fat monster making your stomach jiggle.

Where there is belly fat, there will likely be fat in other areas. Even if it isn't obvious to begin with, it's the start of an unfolding process that will likely spread beyond the belly for most folks. To halt this process in its tracks, you need to address lifestyle habits.

The good news is that once you start improving your dietary habits, exercising regularly, and managing your stress, a flatter stomach will soon follow. Hopefully this book has empowered you with the knowledge that **you don't have to be perfect to get rid of belly fat.**

A few common-sense, moderate changes in your eating and exercise habits should be enough to see results. Yes, some sacrifices will probably be necessary too – but when you behold your gorgeous flat belly, waiting to make its debut at the beach, you'll surely agree that the sacrifices were **MORE** than worth it.

The 5 D's

The Five D's are five key steps which help me to hang on, even when hunger, emotions and circumstances push me to give up. Take your time and put these to practice thoroughly as I know that they will help you a lot.

* **DECIDE** that you are through with the old way of things. Look at the goals that you have related to your health, weight and eating. Resolve in your heart-of-hearts that you **ARE** going to follow through - <u>no</u>

<u>matter what</u>. Draw an imaginary line that ends your old way of eating and relating to food, health and wellness, and become totally willing to take the action to change **<u>PERMANENTLY</u>** – one day at a time.

* **DEFINE** the type of life that you want to have as a result of your leaner physique. Look at the new avenues, activities and relationships you want to engage in as you move forward.

So, as of now, (*if you haven't done so already*) mark that calendar and decide when you intend to start with this fat-burning process. If you have truly defined the type of life that you want for yourself, then moving forward with your weight loss and health-improvement goals is an absolute must. And I'm not talking about tomorrow, next week or next month. I am talking about **RIGHT HERE AND RIGHT NOW!**

* **DECLARE** to your close friends and family that you are through with being overweight and toxic and that you will be implementing some changes during the next months to lose fat. Tell them that you will **<u>NO</u>**

<u>**LONGER**</u> be indulging in junk food and that you do not wish for it to be offered. The purpose of this step is to give you some immediate accountability with people that know you. You do not, however, have to disclose your plans to everyone. Disclose it only to immediate family members, of course... people that you trust and you know will not judge or try to put banana peels in your path.

You may not realize it, but there are people who will resent that you are taking action to get a hold of your life and health. Be aware and don't let them bring you down!

* **DESIGNATE** a specific person that you trust and tell him or her specifically what you intend to do and why. Ask this person for support during the process and stay accountable to him or her on a regular basis.

Visit **FitnessThroughFasting.com** and go to the forums where you can give and receive lots of support and motivation. There are tons of online forums dedicated to weight loss. Find one that you feel comfortable in and make it a point to get involved with the community. That alone will help you in more ways that you can imagine. In short, this step is designed so that you can determine which person in your close circle would best be suited to support you in the coming months.

* **DEVELOP** a strong journal where you can put in writing the reasons why it is important **FOR YOU** to reach your fat loss goals. Some examples can be;

weight loss, better health, healing from specific illnesses, more energy and vitality, mental clarity, dropping clothing sizes to a particular size, participating in a certain sport, getting married, dating, wearing a bathing suit you always wanted to, having a flat stomach, getting into your high-school-days clothing etc...

These are personal reasons and are crucial because they mean something **TO YOU**... not to your spouse, children or family... but TO YOU. Yes, our loved ones are an immense source of motivation to get us going, but ultimately we have to do this **FOR OURSELVES!**

I cannot stress enough the importance of keeping a journal. In it, you can write the **dreams and goals that are closest to your heart**. You can write exactly what you want to get out of your weight loss efforts. **And those dreams and goals are the powerhouse of your spirit and mind.** Each time you find yourself weak and wanting to give in, you can pick up the journal and read what you have written.

During those moments of weakness, **<u>REMEMBER</u>** the huge payoff in health and weight loss that you will receive. Learn that "a *life worth living is a life worth recording.*"

ROBERT DAVE JOHNSTON

Other Books by Robert Dave Johnston

How to Lose Weight Fast, Keep it Off & Renew the Mind, Body & Spirit through Fasting, Smart Eating & Practical Spirituality

Volume 1: The 'Permanent Weight Loss' Diet

Volume 2: The Intermittent Fasting Weight Loss Formula

Volume 3: How to Lose 30 Pounds (Or More) In 30 Days with Juice Fasting

Volume 4: How to Lose 40 Pounds (Or More) In 30 Days with Water Fasting

Volume 5: Burn the Blubber; How to Lose Belly Fat Fast, and For Good!

Volume 6: Lose the Emotional Baggage: Transform Your Mind & Spirit with Fasting

Volume 7: How to Break a Fast and Keep the Weight Off

Also by Robert Dave Johnston:

How to Lose Weight & Keep it Off by Transforming the Mind & Behaviors

Volume 1: How to Stick to Your Diet &

Achieve Long-Term (And Permanent) Weight Loss

Volume 2: How to Lose Weight & Keep it Off By Reprogramming the Subconscious Mind

Volume 3: Mental Strategies to Defeat Diet Hunger and Junk Food Cravings

Volume 4: The Cravings Ninja Assassin

Volume 5: How to Cheat on Your Diet (And Get Away With It)

Detoxify Your Body, Lose Weight, Get Healthy & Transform Your Life

Volume 1: The 10-Day 'At-Home' Colon Cleansing Formula

Volume 2: Bug Off! A 30-Day Parasite, Liver, Kidney Detox & Weight Loss Plan

Volume 3: Lose 30 Pounds (Or More) in 30 Days with Intermittent Fasting & Coffee Enemas

Don't forget to check the articles and growing health community at: FitnessThroughFasting.com

Rob's first work of horror/fiction has

just been released.

King of Pain – A Journey to Hell & Back through the Mind's Eye Volume 1 – The Descent

Made in the USA
Las Vegas, NV
15 November 2023

80880084R00090